WUTAB

NAZERWAY

Paul Nazer

ISBN 978-1-78280-136-8

Publisher Paul Nazer

http://www.paulnazer.com

Email:admin@paulnazer.com

Simon Christopher and George

My sons

Without the feeling of love I would not have had the desire to be part of their life and for this need then to motivate me to rebuild my life in this new direction.

Table of Contents

Introduction

Chapter One

What You Think, You Become: Wutub. 3

Chapter Two

Problems. 10

Chapter Three

Life Development Processes 13

Chapter Four

Taking Charge 33

Chapter Five

The Body-Mind Interface. 49

Chapter Six

The Bigger Picture. 72

Introduction

There is no belief system involved in understanding this book. It is a guide to change, and how to stay successful, and poses no mysteries in our personal development, making clear that there is an underlying reason for everything.

Reading these narratives provides only a guide to implementing the knowledge to make the changes you require. The book provides the reasons why it is so difficult to change, explains how to be successful and how to develop the motivation required to achieve anything you feel can enhance your life.

I have written the book for all to understand. My clients regularly say to me, "I knew that already", and give an example from their lives; therefore, in this work I feel I have tied together many loose threads. A client said to me recently, "I feel stupid; I should have worked this out for myself years ago". But then it took me 40 years.

There are many reasons why it is so difficult to make changes in life, and these include the natural processes that keep people trapped in spirals of addiction and psychological and physical illness. This book demonstrates that it is possible to channel these processes to become the person you desire to be, and addresses how, with some simple changes, societies' repetitive problems could be reduced.

As a Cognitive Therapist, I have personal experience of having to make such changes, having had to rebuild my life after becoming severely disabled. I found that an interest in my own personal development led to a desire to help my clients achieve their best outcomes on our respective path-ways to success.

Chapter One

WHAT YOU THINK, YOU BECOME: WUTUB

We are alive.

We have made it.

For better or worse,

Richer or poorer,

Sickness or good health,

Our decisions have been made.

We have made the choices that have led us to evolve into ourselves.

We are prepared to fight and even die for ourselves. It could be for something that has gone horribly wrong, and life is a catalogue of failures. Life could alternatively be highly successful. Life could be mundane.

A strong emotional thought, if repeated regularly, becomes encoded in our cells, because the emotions and visualisations that make up individual fantasies evolve the unconscious. If the situation is repeated, the action we took in response to the feelings generated will then also be repeated because the original action had emotional power. This does not mean that the repeated action is a healthy choice. Actually, by now, we may regret the original choice. Here is ambivalence, here is no preference and here is no intelligence in action: What You Think, You Become: *WUTUB*.

This thought might have a physical response, as in addiction, be it substance dependency, gambling, sex or food. Alternatively, the thought might trigger physiological reactions – problems within the digestive system, height-ened anxiety, speech difficulties or educational needs – or psychological problems; thoughts generating actions that appear in our imagination as impulsive desire. This desire is then triggered in similar or identical circumstances, affecting our hormonal and immune systems.

If our imagination and intelligence are at odds, we pre-dominantly follow the fantasies generated by the imagina-tion and then *WUTUB*.

Human lives are built on our own choices, and these choices are then integrated into the "unconscious DNA" and become the blueprint for the construction of our lives. If you are not happy with your life situation, you might scream at the world, "life is crap". But if life is successful, nothing is said. There is no preference in the unconscious; everything good, bad or indifferent is accepted, including all of your imagination's fantasies. If the unconscious could speak, it would scream at the world, "this is what you asked for". The unconscious is like a slave, working towards what has been perceived as the goal, and we become products designed from our own imagination.

In the process of reading at this very moment, the attention you are directing is derived from your intellect. If you stop for a moment and think about this, you take control of your imagination. As I will explain, it is healthy for you to be in charge of the imagination, and unhealthy for the imagination to be in control.

The choices that affect our lives are based on emotion and the imagination. If the individual's intellect is in "positive mode", then the life outcome is positive. But if, while making the choice, the intellect is controlled by a negative emotional spin, the outcome becomes a lottery. The attention placed on a subject may require use of the intellect, but choices regarding a subject also have other influences. If we experience emotional pleasure from the choices based on this fantasy, the easy option would be the overriding choice.

We view everything through reflections from our unconscious, meaning it is critical to understand this phase of the process. Any belief that we hold is a bias over thoughts generated by the imagination. The fantasies thus evoked by the imagination become the major influence controlling the evolution of every aspect of our lives. Again, our unconscious has no preferences; it simply accepts the choices we make in response to external influences. These influences can emerge from any source, but the emotional choices are the ones that endure. It is not like a choice where you might have several items on display and you are told to pick one; instead, it is a choice that generates an emotional sensation. This can be positive, negative or indifferent, and will then determine the direction in which life will develop. They can be healthy or negative, and at a young age we simply go with the feelings and *WUTUB*.

The sixteenth-century Spanish monk Francis Xavier said, "give me the children until they are seven and anyone may have them afterwards". I fell for a powerful influence at seven years old when my father, not then a Chelsea Football Club supporter, took me to see Chelsea play Blackpool at home. My father pointed out Stanley Mathews and told me the reason we were there: "He is the greatest player you will ever see". I was blind to my father's words but I was enthralled and captivated by the emotions and singing from the Chelsea fans and I remain an avid supporter. My constant nagging about everything Chelsea and collection of memorabilia turned my father into one as well. I, then and now, view every football-related item through a blue haze. Influences of a powerful nature remain, even though there is no preference either positive or negative.

We view facts through a fantasy bias, and the same process encompasses any subject matter. Choices are generally made without being processed by intelligence. If a person with a substance dependency could see where that first-time moment of pleasure was going to lead them, they would not have used the substance a second time, and I have not had a client who would disagree.

It does not matter what promoted the thoughts. It could be the most awful circumstances perpetrated on a child, such as abuse or deprivation. Alternatively, everything in a childhood could be idyllic. The process of building the unconscious is the same. A child could have the best public school education with all its advantages and feelings of empowering superiority. Another child may be educated in a deprived inner-city system. The end result for one would be much more beneficial than for the other. But it finally comes down to an individual's thoughts, no matter what has been foisted on them.

If one person believes they are superior, and another thinks they are inferior, they both arrived at the feeling by making a choice to believe it. It is all about thinking, as *WUTUB*. But it can all be changed. We have within us all a marvellous resource that can drive a person to achieve perfect physical and psychological health and life content-ment, or, if left to life's vagaries, to endure the opposite: a life of misery.

The following explains the processes involved in taking charge of life, gaining personal satisfaction and how this process augments change. The readers' thoughts on these statements are the subject. The terminology is not relevant; instead, how the reader perceives what is written is of the utmost importance in starting to understand how to take charge of and direct your life using your individual intel-ligence. By having control of these processes you are then in charge of the direction of your life both physically and psychologically.

Why are bad habits hard to change?

A person's refusal to do something by saying, "I can't do that", often brings forth the indulgent response, "there is no such word as can't". Another word to describe what is happening is "stuckness". This creates ambivalence and procrastination, which could also be called resistance, stuckness or intractability. It is referred to medically as Cognitive Dissidence, conflicting thoughts not supported by intellect. These are viewed as psychological, but the phenomenon also results in a wide-ranging list of physical illnesses that are seen as psychosomatic. However, our own thoughts can also develop a successful life for us, which then benefits everyone we come into contact with.

Drug and alcohol professionals tend not to use the word "addiction" when addressing clients because labelling is not helpful, and labels can become excuses not to move. Dependency is the most frequently used word, and this can be interchanged with stuckness, which is the natural outcome for any repeated action. While alive we become what we think of as our "Self". What we consider "normal" is difficult to change, which is great when life is perceived to be OK, but when an unwanted element is present we have to overcome this ambivalence. There is a struggle between alternating positive and negative emotions when trying to move away from being stuck, with a competing pull back to the existing "You". This You could be a substance user, an overzealous exerciser or a "problem thinker", and this will affect esteem.

We recognise stuckness when, for example, a person becomes institutionalised. People can become used to any conditions, and institutional stuckness can be psychological, as with a lasting depression, or physical, as with afflictions perceived as psychosomatic or physical, such as conditions caused by bad posture: *WUTUB*. This stuckness then has become our normality; neither good nor bad, simply stuck.

We are stuck with a thought we may have been ruminating on since childhood. A previous behaviour choice can become a continuously repeating pattern of thoughts, such as the process involved in my becoming fanatical about Chelsea Football Club. Any event, repetitive behaviour or thought can become stuck and stay for life. I have been a Chelsea fan for 57 years at the time of writing. All of us can, and do, become stuck. It can be an addiction to a substance, gambling or a particular sexual act; each is a regularly repeating fantasy. We can also become stuck with any thought regarding circumstances we ruminate on in the imagination, which is then returned by the unconscious, at a trigger moment, to the conscious mind as a desire.

Chapter Two

PROBLEMS

Psychological Reasons for Addictions

Extreme belief about a particular viewpoint, which started with fact, then gets a personal spin generated from fantasies. There is no intellectual process involved; the fantasy takes over and we become addicted. This belief can then hold sway, and it can relate to any subject. Bigotry and extremism are examples of beliefs created through stuck thinking. When this happens, intelligence no longer holds sway as if intelligence and fantasy are conflicting, the fantasy will predominate.

Alcohol and drugs, including prescribed medication, can create a physical dependency. This can occur when the body builds up a tolerance to a substance, and increased doses are required to achieve the desired effects and prevent withdrawal symptoms. Therefore, this becomes a chemical and physical stuckness. It is vital if this has occurred to seek help and information from health services. There is also the psychological element of addiction, regularly a major originating cause of the physical addiction, the hardest part to control and the reason why people relapse. The term "addiction" is applied to any circumstance that results in an overriding, compulsive desire, and which instigates the circumstance being regularly repeated.

Psychologically, the amount of pleasure felt is in proportion to a need, so this can then be repeated as a "trigger response" to future similar circumstances. The need that is regularly contemplated becomes overriding and is repeated as your desire in a trigger situation by the unconscious. Given that this is what you have visualised emotionally as a relief from stress and/or anxiety, and ruminated on regularly with self-talk, the particular circumstance is then fixed, stuck and repeated through the imagination and can become a compelling desire.

The same thought process involved in becoming psychologically addicted is found in other conditions. For example, an extreme belief about a particular viewpoint, starting with fact and exacerbated by a personal spin generated from fantasies. There is no intellectual process involved; the fantasy takes over and stuckness, and stuck addictive thinking, follows. It is possible to become a fundamentalist in any subject as any bigotry or ideology can be intensified by regular rumination until it becomes stuck. As stated above, when this happens, intelligence no longer holds sway and the fantasy will predominate.

Reasons for Depression

Your unconscious has developed based on a map devised through emotionally desirable fantasies dating from any time. These fantasies become your unconscious goals, and we regularly find that there may not have been any intellect involved in their formation. The unconscious has been formed from childhood by all those dreams and expectancy of how life will be as the perfect adult. The visualisation is the goal, but the unconscious is plastic and malleable, and goals can change. When a goal has evolved, the desire to achieve it is generated by the unconscious. If these goals are ignored or not sustained, negative mood feelings are generated to encourage you to realign the conscious direction that has been built into your now-unconscious DNA. This *was* what you had desired, but it might not be what you *now* require.

The movement away from this old map generates feelings of being lost or even of madness. This is depression, and if circumstances remain unchanged then the feeling can become stuck; the unconscious and the conscious mind are on opposing paths and negative feelings are in the ascendency. As soon as the conscious direction realigns with the unconscious goal the mood improves, and when the two are in tandem positive feelings are in the ascendency and the goals become achievable. If life changes are necessary, follow steps that help develop new life goals.

These feeling can occur in many circumstances, and there are no boundaries. It simply relates to living differently to your fantasy-built unconscious. Other ambivalent forces involved in sustaining the depression are anxiety and stress. Anxiety is fear and stress is worry, and dissipating either helps weaken depression. In this book, I offer strategies for how to achieve this.

Chapter Three

LIFE DEVELOPMENT PROCESSES

As much as others might want an individual to change, for example, where there is a dangerous level of substance use, and no matter how well-intentioned the advice, tough love fails because the harder someone is pushed the harder they fight back. The individual is more likely to sustain the level of usage or even increase their substance use. Ambivalence reacts according to the power present in an action. Reaction = Action, a result often viewed as resistance to change. It is an evolutionary response and a major survival reaction: *WUTUB*. No one complains when a life is externally perceived as being healthy. Remember, the unconscious has no preference; it constructs everything according to the supplied map. To make changes we need to work with the processes involved in our individual life evolution.

For example, a highly confrontational client had her two children taken into care. She had been told by Social Services that until she changed her lifestyle the situation would not be reviewed. I gave her an explanation of how the influences and her blinkered choices from a young age had brought her to this situation, and that at no time had her choices been considered ones, just the easy options of that particular moment. I explained how it was possible to change by using her intellect to make choices so as not to respond to the fantasy-derived decisions that appear as desires from her dysfunctional past. At the end of our session the client thanked me, saying, "everyone keeps telling me what to do, but you have told me *how* I can do it". Within four weeks the client's life changed completely. Her decisions became choices not of confrontation, but of a reasoned, all-win position, making a positive outcome possible.

Ambivalence is a survival tool, often viewed therapeutically as a curse that stops people changing. People do not seek therapy to change when their lives are satisfactory, meaning the ambivalence is then a positive. Our unconscious has no preference; it generates desires in a given situation to ease anxiety. This might have been an emotional choice, or it could have been a moment of impulsiveness in the past without any thought of consequences. If our unconscious has assigned positive, pleasurable feelings to a specific item, when experiencing a trigger event it then produces a desire to help achieve the goal: *WUTUB*.

You may have had a trigger response to a paranoid feeling to which you have responded in the past by having a drink – be it alcohol, coffee or tea – a cigarette or a cake. You would only have had to feel the pleasure and comfort the substance provided a few times for this to become a trigger response and for the unconscious to produce a desire to repeat the comfort felt before. It does not produce choices for you; it could equally have chosen to drink water, eat an apple or go for a walk. It could produce a desire for heroin, cocaine or cannabis, as there are no unconscious preferences and no intelligence. You have responded to the trigger before, so the desire to repeat this comforting response will arise. When willpower and imagination are in conflict, imagination usually wins.

It has been theorised since the nineties that DNA is the unconscious reason why animals instinctively act as a species from shortly after birth, and have the ability to flee or hide. Many species of birds have their own bonding courting rituals and instinctively build identical nests due to a collective unconscious. Between ten and one hundred trillion cells are generated from the original cell at conception, and all are seeking the best way to survive as they evolve through life. DNA nuclei have as their memory the time in the womb, an emotional memory of security. There are no instructions for a child; choices are made and repeated and, once encoded, DNA forms our world. From the moment of birth, thinking shapes every aspect of our lives. The inherent blueprint genetically passed from our parents is the foundation for our survival. From the beginning, our cells are endlessly malleable and can develop in any way, guided by our emotional visualisations, our fantasies. We psychologically accept our positioning in life.

The normal positioning then for the security of our cell is ambivalent or stuck. One factor that differentiates us from other species is the ability to control our individual evolution. There is no instruction manual for how to make the best choices for individual evolution, so we just accept our position in life: stuck. But it does not have to be like this, as *WUTUB*.

Our response to a given situation could be compared with Russian physiologist Ivan Pavlov's animal experiments on repetition. During the 1890s, Pavlov experimented on getting dogs to salivate, using a bell as a stimulus. Whenever he gave food to his dogs, he also rang a bell. After repeating this a number of times, he rang the bell on its own, which now was causing an increase in salivation. The dogs had learned an association between the bell and the food and conditioned a response. In this manner, we also repeat actions as a conditioned response. Our cells' DNA has no preferences. There is no right or wrong; their existence relates to our individual survival as they are directed individually, and there is no cellular-level intelligence. Cells are malleable, and evolve and form from their genetic foundation according to our thoughts. Our individual intelligence, physical prowess, body shape, health – psychological and physical – looks and personality then evolve. From these factors, *WUTUB* defines our health, wealth and, through this, our happiness.

I had just taken control of my first pub when a guy known to the regulars as "Mad Ivan" arrived. He always stood away from the bar area but would suddenly start shouting, the alcohol lifting a lid, releasing some horror, I guess from the Second World War. He would count, "1-2-3-4-5 line them up bang-bang". As this started, those near the door opened it and I lifted the bar flap before going to eject him, but my partner said to me, "be gentle, he can't help being mad". This became a life changing moment for me when I realised that I had not chosen to be "me" either.

With this thought, I decided I would talk with him the next day. As he was barred from all the other local pubs, I told Ivan he could keep coming into the pub but could only have three pints of the standard beer then leave. After the decree he would keep the tally and would say first, second or third – or last – pint, then leave. After a while he came to sit at the bar and talk to customers, and I now realise he had made an emotional decision to change. Emotional choices only endure because of stuckness.

I know people can make life-altering changes. As individuals, we can all prove this by gaining an understanding of the processes affecting our lives. It is not curing, it is healing by altering previous choices that have over time proved to be misplaced and only exist through misjudged non-selective thinking. Our conscious mind acts on these emotional choices – accepted by the unconscious as our perceived goal – if we do not investigate them. Ambivalence is then stuck, even though the consequences are unwanted. These outcomes could be addiction, obesity, depression, isolation, failing at education or a dysfunctional lifestyle; again evidence of *WUTUB*. This is interpretation by our unconscious, resulting in it producing the map for how we are to evolve as an individual. If the unconscious could speak to us at this moment it would say, "this is what you asked for".

Our cells, with their DNA, have no preferences; there is no right or wrong. There is no time in the unconscious, just the present. The unconscious is continually evolving to give us its perception of our requirements for optimum survival, and no cellular-level intelligence cells form from our emotional thoughts and visualisations. Instead, they build from their genetic foundation. At birth, our DNA programs us to survive by bonding with our mother. At the cellular level is the memory of the safety of life in the womb. The main driver to progress is anxiety over a fear of extinction. Food and protection are required, and if fed regularly and comforted, a child's fear levels are tolerable. Fear translated to anxiety then will be proportionately low. Feeling safe is prevalent.

Encouraging feelings of contentment and safety enable the child to be adventurous. The reality is that there are many reasons why this has not been possible, perhaps due to a busy mother, siblings, work, illness, mental health problems or chemical dependency, meaning the child experiences a higher level of background anxiety. Generally, children want to be good, liked and protected. If parents are consistent, supportive and they themselves have low levels of stress and anxiety, a child can develop while grounded in low anxiety levels. If a child is born into a dysfunctional family where this has not been possible, the child has a higher background level of anxiety and many survival tactics are set in motion. The internal dialogue initiated by these circumstances can last a lifetime: *WUTUB* is underway.

As we have said, there is no right or wrong at a cellular level because cells are busy reprogramming for survival. As there is no cellular-level intelligence, cells are malleable, evolve and form to our thoughts. In this way they build from their genetic foundation, and the birth DNA passes on instructions based on how our predecessors survived.

This covers our early development. Babies learn that by giving a variety of signals they get different responses (e.g., crying, smiling or eye movement). This is instinctive until the imagination, through our emotions and visualisations, takes over. From this point, *WUTUB* is in progress.

Therefore, we might have it all wrong. In many cases anxiety is caused by thinking patterns that date from childhood and the beliefs that developed because of the power we gave our imagination. We can believe that we know what people are thinking. However, if we try to conform to what we believe are others' thoughts, or think we know what others should do with their lives, this dysfunctional thinking leads to a dysfunctional lifestyle: *WUTUB*. If, however, our lives have developed from the belief that our imagination is intelligent, allowing our lives to transcend this fantasy, the result can be positive. Life has no preference. Successful people could have a positive internal dialogue over many issues and still be sabotaging their lives with a misheld belief. In many ways, internal dialogues can either sabotage a life or make it hugely successful. No one complains about stuckness when someone is successful, but the process is the same.

Life is full of opposites. For example, when a person has a strong desire for praise, criticism is hard to accept. If pride has buttressed a person, they can find shame intolerable. If a certain point of view is much-desired, the opposite will be proportionately repellent. A strongly felt emotion can be a precursor for a person to be devastated when ambivalence is forcibly ended. The depths of feelings are proportional to them; for example, the depth of grief felt on losing a loved one is proportional to the amount they were loved. Likewise, a person can be highly successful in a work situation that they enjoy and then have to endure the devastation of retirement. The love for the lost, or the wrenching from a cherished environment; this emotional wrench can form a new ambivalence around grieving when the unconscious experiences a nothingness: an emotional feeling of loss. This depression, in some, will not disperse without shifting the ambivalence.

One client lost a much-loved parent in her teens and became depressed. After this initial depression, throughout her life she suffered further bouts following the loss of something, but often disproportionate to the loss, whether a broken or lost possession, moving home or another death. When working with a depressed client in this category it doesn't matter whether the incident that started the depression was five or twenty-five years ago; the unconscious has developed to keep us evolving depending on an individual's life development. In my experience of working with clients, there often seems to be proportionality between how successful their life is and how difficult they find it to assimilate their loss.

Profound, emotionally held beliefs are often repeated from childhood onwards. If a life has been lived with consistency, especially where there are strong drives for safety and contentment, the unconscious will have no preferences. However, consistency can take many forms. Not always making choices just accepting whatever happens as fate. These responses can take many forms, as an individual might think that is just who they are, and not consider the possibility that they can make changes. Society may deem them beneficial, or they could generally be viewed as anti-social. Whatever the direction taken, the unconscious is stuck and generates the desire to retain the status quo and accept the condition, be it healthy or unhealthy.

As a child, one client had often helped her mother with housework, and was regularly told that she was a natural homemaker and mother. This belief became enshrined and everything was perfect until the birth of her first child when she could not breast feed. From this, years of depression followed and alcohol became a problem. Another client was highly successful in every sphere from childhood and felt a responsibility for his whole family. Then in his forties a severe illness struck, he was unable to adjust to feelings of impotency and used alcohol as a prop. For both of these people the unconscious, enshrined beliefs were contrary to the reality.

Confused messages are generated through the imagination. The break from the normal has no place, while feelings of being lost, or feelings of madness surrounding this feeling of being lost, can stay and proliferate through rumination on the internal dialogue. This is regenerated by the unconscious supplying the desired visualisations and constantly thinking about an event. The unconscious and the conscious mind are not in tandem. These feelings can last endlessly as the unconscious knows no time. Whatever is produced repeatedly, and emotionally visualised, is accepted.

The choices we make determine every facet of our lives. Many choices are made first by our thoughts and imaginations. Some are not based on knowledge, and we have no consideration for the consequences of any actions based on these choices. We only need to think a certain way on a small number of occasions before ambivalence locks in the action. For example, a parent throws a ball, the child fumbles, and the parent says they are "no good at sport". The child accepts this and spends their life not participating in sport. A thought needs only an emotional feeling and a small number of subsequent repetitions for it to be repeated throughout life.

The history of famous sportsmen and women has a common denominator; a parent that is highly encouraging if a child has an aptitude for a sport, with constant reassurance that "you are really good at this". Therefore, *WUTUB*, with the constant thought of, "I am really good at this action". Alternatively, a child struggling with mathematics asks a parent for help. The parent's response is, "I can't do sums", so a common response is to take the easy option; the child thinks, "I can't do sums either". Nevertheless, this thought need only be repeated and throughout the child's life he might think, "I am no good at maths"; when a different reaction would have led to a different, more positive, thought. A child just starting to eat solid food has potatoes, meat and greens on their plate when a sibling says, "I don't eat this green stuff". The easy option is for the child to decide, "I don't eat green stuff either", and if repeated this action may lead to a lifetime of not eating greens. If all present had said that greens are great, a lifetime of healthy eating could have followed.

At no time do the consequences of these actions become

part of the choice. These life-forming choices are repeated constantly throughout a child's development. For example, a juvenile looking at a young adult smoking might think, "they look cool"; the desire to smoke is then prevalent and there is no thought for the negative consequences of smoking.

Choices have been the major component in our development, and these choices have been influenced by decisions generated by our imagination; our intelligence has not been involved. Emotionally based thoughts that we have accepted without understanding the consequences take many forms and can be positive or have many detrimental effects on our lives. The unconscious has no preferences; it is not intelligent. It builds our lives on the emotions and pictures it receives from our thoughts, and these can dictate body shape, ageing and ongoing health.

Feelings and beliefs become embedded in the unconscious, and from this the unconscious directs the construction of our lives. We then view the world and make our judgements through our unconscious, and through these reflections we become ourselves. Often these are not choices made using our rational intelligence, but we declare them as our beliefs. These can be positive or negative, as the unconscious has no preference and no concern for the consequences for our future psychological and physical health.

The choices we make can be imposed due to a wish to conform, take the easier option or follow trends or fashions, or swayed by people who have learned to use the power of persuasion to bypass a subject's intellect by appealing to their emotions. We know the power our thought processes have over our life, but it is not put into context. At this point we have evolved through the choices we have made. These choices become our actions and are encoded into our DNA by our emotional response to them. Our DNA is linear; it starts at birth and ends at death. It knows no time, just this moment, from the development of the first cell and throughout all subsequent cell duplication. Our response to our DNA is an unconscious reaction; it is not intelligent and has no preferences beyond our personal survival. It repeats a response as a desire encoded by a previous emotional choice in a similar situation. This means that our choices make us.

We all have minds, intellect and intelligence. What we do not have are instructions on how to use them to the best advantage in gaining a contented life. Our unconscious has no preferences, leaving the development of life to the vagaries of choices made predominately from the easier options. Negotiating any external factors without using intellect means anything can evolve from these choices, which will then last a lifetime. It is not explained to children how to develop, but it is common to have expectations of them. Imagination is then used to make choices, which has generally evolved from the fantasy of what is required and taking predominantly the easy option. So our intelligence is generally not in the ascendency when it comes to controlling our burgeoning maturity.

Any repeated response to an event that leads to an emotional choice is achieved through emotional repetition encoded in our DNA and repeated back to us as desire; for example, "I love this" or "I hate this". These powerful thoughts become major triggers to an action. What the unconscious perceives as a thought is of the utmost importance in understanding how to take charge and direct our lives using our individual intelligence. By having control of this process, we are then in charge of the direction our life takes.

WUTUB

Unless we can take charge, our lives are a lottery. These choices form our life and remain with us, but are added to and altered by circumstances. The choices are made as if a person was wearing frosted glasses when the easy option is taken. We all survived infancy with a mixture of responses, such as anxiety, stress, love or anger. A response to our DNA encoding can now guide our actions for our entire lives.

We only have to have a thought or perform an act that has any emotional response three or four times and it can be there for life. A trap snaps down over the event and the choice *becomes* our Self; it is fixed and becomes stuck. The difficulty we have in changing is comparable to Newton's Second Law: *The pressure of the reaction equals the pressure of the action.* Terms like determination, willpower, stubbornness and bull-headedness are bandied about, but the reality is that the more someone is pushed to change, an equal and opposite reaction will come into play. This can also occur when we attempt to use our own willpower to push for change. Any encoded belief, positive or negative, is going to prevail most of the time when opposed by willpower.

When willpower and imagination are in conflict,

imagination will win over time. For example, a determination to diet in the morning can be defeated by a regular response to a situation, say a difficult journey, criticism at work, the smell of food and the comfort and pleasure of eating, so willpower struggles. Similarly, for years a response might have been to have a cigarette and a cup of tea. All the years of saying, "I really need a cigarette", and the pleasure felt emotionally at that moment, has become encoded. The automatic response to a situation is a picture in the mind's eye conjuring the feeling of relief. But the unconscious is not an intelligence; it is just doing its job, helping us survive and develop as per our imagination's blueprint. It has no preference.

Why are bad habits, such as psychosomatic ambivalence, being stuck or phobias, so hard to change? It's because they are generated through our unconscious as a means of survival, evolving as we age. At some stage we have visually focused on a situation and there has been an emotional reaction. Sometimes, this results in a person developing a beneficial aptitude. For example, the individual could develop excellence in academics, sport, music, dance or art, an aptitude developed from choices and which has become encoded into the unconscious. This would be as difficult to change as any perceived negative action. So *WUTUB* helps us through life too, because if an event is thought of as healthy our unconscious accepts it as desirable, regardless of how others might view it, because at some time it was a choice we made with emotion.

Self-sabotaging ambivalence can keep us stuck psychologically and physically, waiting and hoping emotionally for an external source to bring relief from any particular torment. So because the unconscious is not intelligent, the torment is prolonged. It is not possible to give a picture with emotion to the unconscious of "I don't want this problem" because all that is presented is the problem itself, which is then perpetuated by the desire in our thoughts: *WUTUB*. Time cannot heal an event that is still being perpetuated in the mind.

For example, viruses produce a very powerful response: streaming eyes, runny nose and sore throat. Our immune system is quick and active in responding to our thoughts, and this is an incredibly misunderstood, misused part of human life. We cause misery and prolong illness because we are feeding it the wrong information. Take this simple example: a sneeze could result in the thought, "an irritant, nose cleared out, life carries on". Another person might think, "I'm getting a cold". A repeated emotional picture from the past is then produced, and you may feel angry and think, "I don't want this cold". Next morning, symptoms can appear when there is no virus. Similarly, with hay fever, the sun comes out in spring and sufferers think, "hay fever time again", so the eyes and nose respond to produce the consequences, resulting in flushing the system when no pollen irritant is yet in circulation.

Many illnesses seem to result from an overreaction by the immune system, while too much knowledge about a condition can stop remission occurring. One example is arthritis. Knowledge of possible outcomes results in the patient researching them and emotional ideation, and the problem becomes the only image generated. The visualisation required to aid remission or recovery is a picture of a healthy you. Read the restore point exercise and *WUTUB*: the unconscious produces what is emotionally visualised. When a prognosis of death or severe disability is offered, a picture is generated perpetually by an internal dialogue, determined by a person's understanding and perception of the course or the outcome in the mind: *WUTUB*. If a patient's thoughts are negative regarding outcomes, this, to the unconscious, becomes the goal.

In the Western world we are incredulous that people believe in and react to voodoo and black magic, yet at the same time we know that people's health can improve while receiving placebos during drug trials. In the complementary alternative medicine industry, people claim remarkable results from a cross section of unproven alternative therapies. A person is seeking help to change if they sit down and talk to a person with some expertise. Some part of any healing or life changes can be put down to *WUTUB* in some cases as these therapies can provide a positive result if an emotional belief has occurred; in essence, the psychological element of the illness can be healed with a movement away from ambivalence.

If a person is perceived as an expert by a client seeking help to change, and if both are motivated to work towards a goal, the balance of probabilities is a positive outcome. Tests have shown that the stronger the impact the expert makes, the stronger the belief in achieving the goal. It is the belief in achieving that moves people on from being stuck. The more you emotionally believe you are being successful, and visualise this, the better your chances of achieving your goal. The unconscious can only accept what is presented to it. Addictions, psychological disorders and physical illness all involve the *WUTUB* effect to some extent, especially regarding any long-lasting symptoms, which can be as many and varied as peoples' thoughts. The following are examples of the processes involved:

We unwittingly create a significant part of long-term dependency and possible symptoms of a fatal illness ourselves.

Addiction and dependency are hard to break away from because they derive from a repeated emotional desire.

If we dwell on any part of our personal existence in our imagination, whether painful or pleasurable, our unconscious will assist us in achieving a powerful emotional belief.

Because the unconscious is not intelligent and has no preference, it helps us achieve and provides us with emotional desires to keep us on our correct path.

The depth of emotional relief caused by a decrease in anxiety levels when a person first uses a substance, and the comfort and pleasure felt, is proportional to the depth of any burgeoning dependency.

For example, a smoker may gain relief from stress when starting smoking, but it could stem from something as simple as feeling accepted and more grown up. The emotional picture of the belief that he is feeling stress relief is accepted by the unconscious. Now, any trigger in the same situation that then occurs signals a picture of desire to the unconscious, matching the original emotional choice to the current situation. It means we receive a message signalling a desire to end the current anxiety. If a picture of a cigarette is generated, it relates to what has been repeatedly requested: "I really need a cigarette". Resisting the desire leads to more stress, thus increasing desire.

Perhaps at a certain time of day there is a break, say after a meal, and the unconscious, having been repeatedly informed of a desire, will perhaps generate an inappropriate, repeated emotion linked to a related event that has previously caused stress. As the unconscious is primed for your survival, the perceived need embedded within it is that this is necessary to exist. So even though the intelligence may be screaming, "cigarettes are killing me", where there are conflicting thoughts the imagination will predominate and triumph.

Psychological symptoms caused by ambivalent thinking can occur following an event that is outside the norm. The negative thought is then in mind for an extended period, causing a low mood. *WUTUB*: if there are no preferences then the causing event can be resolved. But the low mood can remain because time does not always heal; *WUTUB* can occur and ambivalence and the low mood can stay for years. This may eventually be diagnosed as clinical depression. The same process can apply physically, as a person can become ill with a virus when all the symptoms of the illness are protracted and focused upon. *WUTUB* is in operation because if we cannot form a picture of "I don't want the virus", the only picture that occurs is "I want the virus". So protracted illness is what you asked for and continuously ask for, this is ambivalence, and the unconscious constructs life based on the emotional need of "what is asked for". The body can display symptoms of an illness long after the original causal event has been rectified. This stuck thinking naturally occurs all the time, and can be reinforced by a causing event.

I listened to a radio programme on which a doctor from the USA talked about having to live with arthritis and her actions, in the form of consulting with the best experts. She had tried a variety of medications, all with little benefit. I felt the approach was failing because she was continually thinking about the ailment, its course and the possible outcome. The emotional response and visualisations this thinking would evoke prompted the unconscious to respond to this blueprint because *WUTUB*. It is as if she was asking for the arthritis inflammation.

One client referred for an alcohol problem was a career woman, then in her mid fifties. She had some arthritis and was having difficulty accepting that she was ageing. I explained about *WUTUB* and suggested trying the Restore Point exercise discussed in the next chapter. Our sessions finished with the client in remission; by taking charge of her thought process she was then in control of her life. Severe prolonged events can result in fixed thinking and can stop remission. The non-preferential unconscious would construct a healthy life if the emotions and visualisations it received signalled the best attainable health. But if the underlying thought relates to death, even if life is being lived in what is viewed as a positive way, the actions on the surface only mask the underlying emotional belief. If a person becomes an "expert" in their illness and its likely course, and is regularly checking for signs of the illness developing, then *WUTUB*. It does not matter if all external actions are positive; it is the underlying belief that guides development. No matter what the external actions are, if they are suppressing a person's emotional belief then *WUTUB*, meaning the imagination will predominate.

Chapter Four

TAKING CHARGE

The Restore Point Exercise

The unconscious knows no time; it accepts visual and emotional stimulus – fantasies – as if occurring in the present by reliving a time when the undesired event was not occurring. The unconscious and conscious minds are then in tandem, equilibrium is restored and the psychosomatic aspect of an illness can be resolved. The "Restore Point", reached by shifting the psychosomatic side of an illness, allows people to find that the illness no longer exists and that the condition had been resolved through natural means. This does not require any faith or belief; if you give the unconscious a happy, cheerful feeling it will give back positive desires.

Whether physical or psychological, if the mind has dwelt on anything for an extended period of time any condition can become stuck by ruminating on the stressor. A trauma can interrupt a life in this manner. However, the Restore Point can involve short exercises to allow a life to return to normal and out of the negative ambivalence. I have explained this exercise to people over several years.

Some of my clients have been depressed for years after a single event, sometimes in excess of twenty years.

Examples include the tragic death of a much-loved person, divorce, leaving an adored home, serious illness, a work situation and a professional having to endure an excessive amount of stress over a prolonged period and finally having a breakdown, never being able to return to work. They had all become stuck, unable to move on from the trauma and emotionally fixated on the ending: *WUTUB*. All of the positive experiences that had occurred before were lost to the unconscious, and everything was viewed with a negative spin. Positive thoughts could never prevail, thus causing a permanent background of a low mood.

This feeling can be countered. Pick a time before the event by recalling happier times. See yourself as being healthy, talking to people; see it all in a bright light. Remember cheerful conversations, celebrations, meals, parties, walks in the garden, decorations in the home, old furniture, toys and cars of that time. See yourself playing your favourite sports. Look at old photographs. Watch films you enjoyed, play the music of that era. Think of a holiday with friends and loved ones. Live at this time for a week. This often provokes dreams of people and events long-forgotten; to the unconscious you are there and it causes an adjustment, lifting the brake of stuckness. The unconscious cannot comprehend loss. Just try to recall an object or person you no longer have; all it does is evoke a picture of the subject, and the emotions generated do not match the picture generated. Confusion ensues when what was once a pleasurable picture is viewed with sadness. This then becomes depression, and using the Restore Point exercise helps removes the confusion.

The Value of Goals

Without a goal, life is like a rudderless ship whose destination is left to the vagaries of the elements. A goal provides the stimulus in motivation. Now imagine a destination with a walled route; set off to get there and you will be successful. This is how a goal works. There might be every kind of distraction from outside, but by focusing on the destination the unconscious will generate the desire to achieve, instead of generating distracting thoughts and temptations.

Goals are of the utmost importance in our lives. Indeed, you might be working towards one at the moment. Unfortunately, many of them are negative. We may not realise that where we are in life is the result of a goal, but one created by dysfunctional thoughts and beliefs. People can go through life full of envy, jealousy, paranoia and complaints. If this is what you are ruminating on then misery develops: *WUTUB*. The goal held deep within us might be to conform or to be a rebel, to be part of an ethical society or to be a criminal. These goals could have been formed without the use of the intellect, and exist in the unconscious where there are no preferences. Without goals we could end up drifting in life, always looking outwards for a mother figure or other carers to nurture us.

From birth, it is natural to have developed a strong feeling of reliance and to look outward to find psychological and physical health. The overriding desire can be to wait for the world to produce the answers. This then means the unconscious does not produce the desire to self-motivate, which then becomes a map for the unconscious to produce the asked-for lethargy. Helplessness means there is nothing for the unconscious to achieve except assist with a personal continued desire for hopelessness. No ambition to achieve, and instead accept ailments, illness and bad health; there is no sense of self-esteem, just acceptance. Instead, we look to external interests, for example TV soaps, sports, games, social networks, alcohol and drugs, seeking the excitement to stimulate adrenaline release. This often leads to crime, gambling and promiscuity; without goals we are lost, drifting in the world.

Once there is a goal, everything becomes possible. By being focused, the unconscious helps to achieve positive endings instead of producing the desires that lead to distractions. If a goal is embedded in the mind, negative emotional drives are not generated, being replaced by the desire to achieve the goal. First comes the decision regarding what you want to achieve. To do this, visualise an overall picture of the future, such as employment or lifestyle, then break this down into smaller components, for example, type of home, type of area, transport, pastimes or hobbies. Keeping the component parts reasonably achievable will help provide motivation for the next level. The same process can be used to help with motivation for smaller goals.

Take a client – a business person – recovering from alcohol dependency. Having to enter a situation where alcohol is available for the first time scared him. But fear evaporates when you face up to it. By visualising the event and deciding what actions to take, the goal is just to survive without drinking. First, he would visualise leaving the premises, feeling pleased that he had been successful. So in breaking this down, he will only drink soft drinks, he will talk to people and if pressed tell them he is not drinking and finally he would leave immediately if tempted to drink alcohol. Success is earned by visualising these actions and saying repeatedly to himself, "this is what is going to happen". This can become a huge motivator because until then the thought of going through the rest of life not drinking and socialising seemed daunting or even impossible. But this small success becomes a major step in a new journey.

In goal setting there is a need to focus on the outcome, as only thinking about the start and the delivery leaves room for doubt and fear. But visualising completion and hearing the congratulations will result in success: *WUTUB*; the intellect is in charge. For example, lying in bed thinking about ploughing the furrow required for this year's potato crop is daunting; visualising autumn's huge crop and next winter's food motivates action. Create the "big picture" of what you want to do with your life and then break this down into smaller targets that you need to achieve to reach the larger life goals. Once you have your plan, start working on it. Work down to the things that you can do in five years, followed by next year, next month, next week and today. Having a goal at all times is the mindset of successful people. Once a goal is in place, it is important to realise *WUTUB* and that the unconscious is constructed predominately from the imagination. Starting to take charge of your life is necessary to establish the difference between the intellect and the imagination. Although this seems obvious, I have seen clients struggle for several weeks to tell the difference; it is vital to contemplate understanding this difference.

Understand that you cannot read others' minds, and that the thoughts of others have no place in your life. I regularly explain this to clients by saying, "look at me. I am thinking about you. I think you are wonderful and love you". Changing track, I then say, "I am thinking you are rubbish and hate you". I add quickly, "my thoughts about you don't matter at all in your life. What is important to you and to your unconscious are your feelings. If you love or hate someone".

We saw earlier that the unconscious is constructed from our emotional thoughts and visualisations. So to get the maximum assistance to attain a goal the intellect must be in control of any choices made. The relationship of thoughts to emotions takes some understanding. For example, you might start the day in a low mood and a negative emotional state. You look in the mirror in the morning and the mirror says, "your life is a mess, you are useless, unappealing, a failure". During the rest of the day, everything will be viewed with a negative spin. Even small positives will be transformed into negatives, and by the end of the day nothing positive has been achieved in terms of attaining the goal. But if you begin the next day in a positive mood, the mirror says, "you are marvellous, good looking, everyone's friend, a high achiever". Throughout the day, nothing is negative, life is great and there is a positive spin everywhere. This is a day of movement towards the goal.

These two examples are, of course, normal in the roller-coaster of life. But by understanding the process and putting intelligence in charge, the morning look in the mirror will result in you saying, "this is what's going to happen today, no longer controlled by life's vagaries; every day is controlled by getting closer to the goal".

Controlling Thoughts

Although thoughts make up our emotional feelings, our emotions control our thoughts. Think about this and read the following analogy:

Imagine two locked filing cabinets in your torso. One is full of negative thoughts, the other full of positive thoughts. The keys to unlock them are your emotions. When you are in a positive emotional state the only thoughts you can have will be positive. This means any negative thoughts will then have a positive spin. When the negative filing case is opened, all thoughts are negative and all life events are given a negative spin. You need to learn how to choose your emotional state. It is only a thought that determines it at first, so it is necessary to check which state you are in at the start of this exercise. Get in the habit of checking your emotional state and knowing you can change it.

Exercise

Print a list of recent positive achievements that make you happy (for me, I just need to think of Chelsea winning the Champions League!). For example:

1. Reading this and doing exercises to help achieve the desired goal
2. You are alive
3. You are cognitive
4. Your children
5. A recent meeting or party you enjoyed
6. An enjoyable TV programme
7. An enjoyable concert
8. Your home
9. Family and friends
10. A recent holiday

Anything that leaves a happy feeling puts you in positive state. Unlocking the positive filing cabinet will change your emotional state so that, after a while and with practice, you can simply think, "click fingers, change emotions and it will occur".

Stress & Thought Stopping

Worry is stress. Repetitive thinking keeps people trapped with many conditions, and stopping these spinning thoughts is crucial in keeping depression at bay and overcoming dependencies. I was explaining the concept of Thought Stopping to a client recovering from long-term heroin use. He said that for twenty-five years he had just one thought: "Get money, get drugs, get out of my head". Thoughts become invasive with regards self-esteem. Clients have found negative thoughts perpetuating and follow the pattern of, "they think this about me" and "they think I am this". This is generated by the imagination, with no intellect involved.

To take charge, it is first necessary to catch yourself thinking. Thought Stopping and thought control have been practised to help achieve spiritual aspirations since early times. People find numerous ways of trying not to hear their negative internal dialogue, which is often detrimental to good health. It is all just thoughts, and very little of it proves to be factual. It is a form of mind games that started as children and which has been perpetuated by being ruminated on ever since, with only the characters changing.

Thought Stopping is to catch and stop individual thoughts and then use intelligence to decide which thoughts to accept. People have found this useful for dissipating self-harming thoughts and dispersing phobias and compulsive behaviours. It has also helped people overcome speech impediments. I always start with it to assist relapse prevention when working with substance abuse clients or in any situation driven by thoughts, generated through the imagination by the unconscious, whether physical or psychological.

We can only have one thought process in action in the mind at a given moment, and if intelligence is in operation, no invasive thoughts stemming from the imagination can intervene. It is important to understand that you must not think in negatives, we cannot think in terms of "not" or "don't". We would want this only to conjure up a picture of the undesired item: "I don't want to drink alcohol", the only picture is alcohol; "I must not eat that doughnut", the only picture is the problem, the doughnut. However, a simple strategy, such as reading, stops the imagination in its tracks. Any object on which attention is placed keeps out the imagination.

Clients regularly make statements about why they think they are being held back in life, placing the blame on others who could now be long in the past or even no longer a tangible part of their life. These beliefs are only in their heads and have no basis in reality. Instead, understanding repetitive thought patterns, what triggers them and what can stop them can change a life. The imagination is wonderful, and often a precursor for intellectual discovery and achievement. But to be successful it is necessary for the intellect to be in charge. If the imagination is controlling a life, the emotional state of any particular moment can cause any kind of excess or potentially harmful choices. The intellect has to be the decision-maker.

Exercise

Here is a simple exercise that demonstrates how thoughts can be controlled.

Go to a comfortable place. Take some deep breaths and relax.

Then in your imagination go alongside yourself and visualise looking into your mind at the point where thoughts are generated.

Keep looking, and when any thought appears say, "STOP".

There is now no thought development.

This is the start of learning to stop thinking.

If there is a regular invasive thought, you could put a rubber band on either wrist, snap the band when catching a thought and say, "STOP".

After working in this way for a time, clients often come up with their own way of stopping thoughts.

Case Study

I explained the process to a female client from a hostel for the homeless who then came up with her own method. At first she felt I was on her shoulder telling her what to do and when to do it. However, the voice changed and became her own, and finally she no longer responded automatically to negative thoughts. They were no longer generated in response to a particular trigger, and new positive thought patterns came to predominate and became the normal response.

One of the hardest choices when selecting thoughts is moderation; but *WUTUB*, and the unconscious and conscious moving in tandem become an unbeatable team. Self-motivation in this way becomes the ultimate solution therapy. Solution therapies are generally long-term and work first by changing individual damaging thoughts and behaviours. This type of therapy has one solution for all circumstances, which is for a person to take complete control of their life and no longer follow old, unwanted, unconscious repetitive thoughts and behaviours.

Self-Talk

Self-talk is a very powerful tool for change, as what we say to ourselves – our ruminations – builds our lives. Talk must be positive and clearly defined. There can be no "ifs", "maybes" or "buts", as every statement followed by a "but" is flawed, while regular "but"-sayers destroy self-esteem. There is a true saying that everything that comes before a "but" is a lie.

There are some very powerful self-talk words. "Can" for native English speakers is the permission word built into the unconscious from infancy as a mother says, "you can do or have that item". When encountering a stuck moment say, "I can do this". "Quickly" is another word with a powerful connotation, while the word "love" creates emotion. I have given this suggestion to many people in a variety of circumstances. During post-natal depression the mother does not feel bonded to her child. If the mother repeats, "I love you" silently to herself while thinking of her child, this can be resolved. Families, for a variety of reasons, can become fragmented, and this technique helps with bridge building by changing your own feelings. The retorts of others are no longer viewed through a negative haze.

In addition, I have had clients who are excessively reserved or have just relocated, and when talking about their inability to make new friends often say, "they don't like me" or, "they think I'm standoffish". I explain that these are only their own internal thoughts, and that they are, in their imagination, thinking they are reading the others' minds. By changing your internal dialogue you change everything;

we all make our own personal world, and I have suggested that in a social situation they say to themselves, "I really like you", adding the name of the person they would like to befriend. *WUTUB* is in action in these circumstances, where we change our view of others by changing ourselves. As explained, our emotions generate our thoughts and, as with the example of the filing cabinets in your torso, when a person is perceived through love it gives a positive spin to our thoughts about them, and your perception of their thoughts is then positive.

Anxiety

Without this we would not move forward in life. Fear starts at birth through thinking, "is mother/carer coming? Am I going to be fed, cuddled and comforted?" There is a need to feel safe in this new environment. Without the appropriate anxiety motivating us in our development we would not begin rolling, crawling, walking or talking. We would not have developed the desire to please, be a good child or earn attention. The imagination begins guessing at what is evolving in life using fantasy; learning to use intellect to survive is driven by the need for food and safety. How these needs are met defines early anxiety levels. If these needs are met then there is little anxiety; if not met then there is a proportionally high anxiety level: *WUTUB.*

Clients often display high anxiety levels, are unable to relax and sit rigidly like a parrot on a perch, while their breathing pattern tends to be very shallow. The trillions of cells in our body remain tense while anxious. The message that the body is safe is transmitted by the breathing pattern, and a couple of yoga-type breaths send the signal that everything is OK, and a regular breathing pattern ensues. The reduction in anxiety from this alone is enormous.

Case Study

A client who had experienced a torrid childhood arrived for therapy sessions in very formal clothes. He had undergone extensive counselling focussing on his traumatic childhood; he understood the reasons for his anxiety and why he responded to repetitive triggers by self-medicating via heavy alcohol consumption. At the end of our first session I demonstrated a yoga breath and asked him to practice this over the coming week in a safe place at home.

People who have used large amounts of substances over prolonged periods find suddenly relaxing without the substance can cause feelings of panic. During the following sessions, the feeling that he was going to run any second dispersed and we worked at Thought Stopping and Taking Control. As time went by his clothing became more casual. At the end of our sessions the client said that one morning he arose and in the mirror appeared a person he had not seen before. He felt his previous formal style was a mask and a form of protection from reality.

Exercise

I give some clients an exercise to go with their wristbands and act as a continuous reminder.

When reaching a door, snap the band and think the words: Calm, relaxed, in control.

CALM: take a breath

RELAX: exhale slowly, feeling your body relax

IN CONTROL: check the mind is clear

Do this every time you use a door.

This "looking into the mind" exercise is about taking control away from the imagination and can also be a powerful aid to falling asleep quickly. If there are any stressful thoughts, make sure you have done as much with them as possible and put down a full stop for the night. Start breathing consciously and, when feeling relaxed, look into your mind. Stop any thought appearing by counting down from twenty and inserting the word sleep at every count: 20, sleep, 19, sleep, 18, sleep… and good night.

Exercises are a great motivator; they work by enabling us to take charge of life's processes and stopping the imagination controlling us.

Relapse Prevention

Psychologically, all the desire invested in a substance that has been ruminated on as a way of relieving a particular stressful time has acted as a diversion activity at a "trigger moment" that occurs whenever a person has concerns or feelings of anxiety. The amount of pleasure felt is in proportion to satisfying a need, so this can then be repeated as a "trigger response" in future similar circumstances. The need that is ruminated on becomes stronger, meaning the demand is repeated by the unconscious. In desiring it repeatedly, it then integrates into your self-talk. This could take the form of "I really need a drink/joint/fix/cake/sex/pain/bet".

A relapse due to the emotional response to a situation involving a repeated behaviour or behaviours from the trigger may be quite trivial. It could be a moment of low self-esteem caused by an imagined slight if, in the past, the way to handle this was to use a substance. It may no longer be a responsive need for an actual substance, and may now be a behavioural reaction, generating a desire in the imagination. No intelligence is involved until anger is felt at this moment of now presumed weakness. This is the crux of relapsing, that intellect is not involved until the realisation that a calamitous relapse has occurred and self-recrimination starts. The patient could have been through this many times, and the coping mechanism is to relapse into old psychological behaviours. There has not been any intellectual pondering on how to recover the status quo, just thoughts of recrimination and blame for the perceived weakness.

All this is relevant to relapse prevention. We need to understand the choices we make, how to recognise triggers and how not to respond to them. This is the reason people need to take charge of thought processes at an early stage. By using Thought Stopping and taking control of your emotional state you gain control of your life, and then anything becomes possible. Your intelligence is in charge, meaning you can make healthier choices.

Chapter Five

THE BODY-MIND INTERFACE

The medical profession uses terms like placebo (positive health change without apparent reason) and psychosomatic (illness without apparent cause), even though medical science does not provide an answer or explanation. But there is a huge amount of anecdotal evidence to prove that the mind affects the body. The process of *WUTUB* applies to the psychosomatic aspects of illness, which can be explored and used for therapeutic benefit.

There is a polarity between the placebo or psychosomatic effects that result from thinking, followed by the stuckness of the outcome, and either can occur with any ailment after a few weeks of rumination, allowing the unconscious to take over. This becomes what you appear to desire; the unconscious cannot respond to conscious desire, as in thinking, "I don't want this", so the picture evoked becomes the goal.

When a drug is prescribed at the start of an illness, no psychosomatic or placebo effect is envisaged. But if the patient is thinking about the complaint and the pain, and worrying, this generates anxiety and fear about the outcome and depression becomes connected to the malady. As time passes, thought is given to it, there is rumination with emotion, and the unconscious produces what is being asked for.

If the patient is not improving then medication may be increased and with time all becomes stuck. The condition could now be entirely psychosomatic; essentially, it is a "stuckness" thought. It may or may not be a reality, as either the placebo or psychosomatic effect could be dominant. The unconscious and conscious would then require realigning to restore the former status quo, or a life adjustment made so that the unconscious accepts a new reality and life then can evolve a new "normality". The illness now might be in a different phase, or no longer exist, but in any prolonged illness the malady becomes stuck based on the imagination's ideation.

Medication

To gain the most benefit from medication the unconscious needs to be working towards the same goal. If the thought is, "this is not working" or "this is not going to work" then a conflict results because the unconscious belief is that the treatment will fail. However, the placebo effect can be understood by looking at the *WUTUB* process.

If a medical practitioner in experimental conditions has a strong positive presence then the patient is more likely to have a positive response. Similarly, if the medical practitioner gives a negative impression then the medication may not produce the same result. If a Tom Cruise lookalike says, "you are going to get better" you might be more likely to do so than if a Quasimodo clone says, "all is well". If a person is prescribed a drug to treat a condition but thinks it is not helping, the drug might not be so beneficial. This means that the unconscious must be in tandem with the conscious self. This accords with the suggestion by Victorian therapist and personal development guru Emile Coue to recite, "EVERY DAY, IN EVERY WAY, I AM GETTING BETTER AND BETTER" when taking medication.

The majority of amputees are thought to experience the feeling of having a phantom limb at some time. Having lost something that is part of your being makes it impossible not to remember it, so even while thinking, "I have lost this limb" the only picture generated is that of the limb, so to the unconscious it may still exist. There is now another process at work. When a person suffers prolonged backache, or any persistent pain or condition on which they have ruminated, the constant thinking about it in the unconscious is as an emotional desire. There is no picture for the thought, "I don't want this bad back". I once witnessed a group of extreme back pain sufferers arrive for a week's physiotherapy and training. The participants arrived in wheelchairs, with walking frames or crutches, but after five days they were all engaged in full-on aerobics.

Every prolonged illness has a psychological impact and it would be, I feel, common to think of death as synonymous with cancer, and for the word cancer to predominate the mind. *WUTUB*: if the imagination and our intelligence are in conflict, eventually the imagination will prevail. Even when using tactics to avoid negative thoughts, the underlying thought remains. Many people with this type of diagnosis decide to make the most of the time left to them. The external view might be "why not", it is everyone's own choice, looking at it from the *WUTUB* viewpoint. But if the underlying thought is death and the conscious thought is fight, the unconscious very often wins; for the best outcome the unconscious needs to be programmed for living and the immune system primed for fighting towards this aim.

WUTUB and the Illness Mindset

For quick relief you can use the Restore Point tactic, then build a picture of yourself being healthy and superimpose this thought over any negative emotions. This tactic is to encourage the immune system to continue its work, as in *WUTUB*. Think of the future, and how you would like your life to develop. Never let that dark thought dwell in the mind. Do not defiantly play mental games with the thoughts; always see yourself as alive. You can only have one thought at one time, so visualise a positive future.

When facing serious illness you need your immune system to work towards achieving good health, and for this to occur the emotional thoughts must be focused on a healthy future. I showed one client with a chronic bad back how to move the pain outside of his body, and he left saying, "it's incredible!" But the following week he reported it only lasted until the next morning. I asked if he had used the self-hypnosis again but he said no, it was a waste of time if it was just going to come back. Another client stopped working towards change because her wristband broke. This is another example of the power of ambivalence, stuckness institutionalised by life. Of course, this is natural because it helps us to survive in general life. To move from ambivalence needs delicacy of movement, as moderating ambivalence cannot be achieved with force. If it were possible to change by force, we could end depression, ME, addiction and backache by torturing people! We know this has the opposite effect, as for every action there is an opposite reaction.

Healthy Mindset for Conditions

Depression

Unipolar depression, sometimes termed exogenous depression, is caused by life events rather than being inherent or endogenous. This can cause a low mood or ambivalence, and there can be many causes. Treatment is often sought when a person is emotionally stuck in a low mood condition. Examples of causes are a change in life that is out of the ordinary, or an extended stress that becomes a part of life and is accepted by the unconscious as the new normality: *WUTUB*. This then is depression.

For a quick change of mood use the Restore Point exercise. This helps readjust emotional memories and enables a different thought pattern that can reconnect to the past. For long-term control, look first at anxiety reduction breathing exercises. Do not let the mind start spinning; use the techniques described to say, "STOP". Don't leave or put off doing something. If you know you have proceeded as far as possible at that time, put a mental full stop down; don't entertain any thoughts on the subject.

M.E.

Myalgic Encephalopathy, Chronic Fatigue Syndrome and fibromyalgia represent the physical equivalent of depression; by enduring physical discomfort, a physical ambivalence or stuckness arises when suffering from a prolonged illness. Feelings become stuck due to the imagination constantly ruminating on the symptoms. This is surrounded by emotional anguish: *WUTUB*; it becomes stuck, and the unconscious – through the imagination – and the internal voice present what is perceived as desired. The unconscious then provides what is being visualised regularly and emotionally. I encourage the use of Restore Point to consider some point in time before the illness. This is meant to break and defuse messages generated and repeated by the imagination, to regain some emotional control and begin then to view life in light of today's reality. The original illness that started the thought process, although prolonged, could have long been cured, and what remains is the stuckness of thought. It must be unjammed to enable the release of the brake restraining you.

The Restore Point helped one client who had been on medication and not worked for six years. He had also been hospitalised for tests, all to no avail. After just one week of using Restore Point his life began again by returning the imagination to the positive state that existed before the trauma intervened. Once there is movement, symptoms no longer exist. Your body doesn't want to give discomfort, it is simply responding to your thinking. There is no sense of time in the unconscious, so by switching the circumstances using emotional visualisations, your life resumes from your fantasy and if you are pleased and happy with this it stays; this is also stuckness.

Type-two Diabetes and Metabolic Syndrome

These conditions may have an element of DNA or ethnic background, but not always. All prognoses are ultimately affected by lifestyle choices. The word "choices" involves a high degree of complicity. If you follow the process described you can understand that the choices made by sufferers were predominately blind ones, with only one option. For example, eat high carbohydrate, highly plea-surable, food, ruminate on the new preference and strongly desire quickly digestible food that gives a carbohydrate high. The only choice really was whether or not to eat the instant, pleasing food.

Of course, there might have been different choices made if the picture also alternated with obesity, blindness, ampu-tation, arthritis, cancers, cardiovascular diseases, skin and hair problems and learning difficulties. If the original choice had been between the above and even more ailments, or a moment's pleasure, it might have been different. But many people form a reliance, a dependency on a high-starch, high-sugar diet. We all regularly hear people say – because of stuckness – "I can't do without a certain food". If this is stuckness, after three or four days of a healthy diet the fog starts lifting from the mind and the choices become the healthy ones, not driven by repetitive desires originating from childhood.

Set a goal and practice Thought Stopping, learn to control your emotions and you can then control choices. Read about relapse prevention, do the Restore Point exercise, construct a You that you desire to be, so that when there are any temptation moments you can substitute a picture of the desired You. *WUTUB*: healthy.

Eating Disorders: Weight Loss

Children might be "comfort fed" by parents perhaps because they have other distractions or are overweight themselves. Comfort foods tend to be high in carbohydrate, and the child's view of himself comes to be one of being overweight. Early concerns might be placated by comfort eating, meaning the emotional picture becomes one of worrying about the weight. The thought must be, "I want to lose weight, I don't want to be fat", because the unconscious has no preference, it generates a desire to develop what is asked for and return you to this unwanted goal of being overweight.

A life map of continuing obesity might consist of the conflict between the conscious mind not wanting to be overweight and the unconscious desire for obesity. The unconscious will predominate and win. Great determination might be used to lose weight, but unfortunately in the unconscious background the desire is for obesity; this is what was desired and unconsciously asked for.

The unconscious generates a desire for food because this was always the manner in which stress was managed. The greater the stress around losing weight the more it can result in a proportional increase in the desire to eat. *WUTUB*: overweight.

To change this spiralling nightmare it is necessary to change the unconscious concept of yourself, the picture that is lodged in the corner of your mind. This new picture can be constructed from any source. It could be from past pictures of yourself looking as you would like to look now, or a composite picture drawn from the media. I would suggest a body of similar stature and an achievable shape. From now on, see this person and smile; be happy when you see it as it is going to be you. When you are out and see a person whose weight and shape is along your desired lines, say to yourself, "yes, that's good", and feel it as being good. Remember, you are not dealing with an intelligence; the unconscious just accepts what is being visualised. If your see a person whose shape was similar to the old you, don't dwell on the picture, turn off your mind and visualise the new picture. The unconscious knows no time. It accepts whatever is repeatedly produced and emotionally visualised.

Now insert this picture into a goal, all the time viewing yourself as being pleased that you will be taking control of your life based on your design, not the old control of the easy choices taken in the past. Use the "new you" picture in fantasies of you attaining your goal and feel pleased. If there are any major trigger moments that need to be navigated, in the mind see the eating response to a trigger. This time, replay it with a new response, and imagine yourself in a bright light, feeling happy. View any trigger response with the healthy option. For a quick start, use the Restore Point exercise, even if it relates to a fictitious time, and keep returning to it with pleasure; remember *WUTUB*, and it will be your choice. These exercises are designed to enable your unconscious to stop producing unhealthy desires by replacing them with healthy influences. With your thinking and willpower working in tandem anything is achievable.

Although Kate Moss and other models are often criticised for their body shape, it gives a glimpse of her mindset regarding retaining her physique when she was maligned for saying, "nothing tastes as good as being skinny". Every time you near a possible eating situation, visualise the new you and keep hold of that thought. Imagination, the very thing that has worked against you, will come to help you with temptation. In my experience, this taking charge is so welcome that it transfers to other areas of life.

Slimming Disorders

The desire to be slim can become overcompensatory. The pictured goal of being thin combines with a conscious drive, and the whole body is geared to attain the goal but this time with a map for malnourishment. The picture generated for the goal is one viewed as desirable; role models could be neighbours, friends, relatives or others, as in this age of mass media there are many influences. Life development could have taken this to an extreme. Body shape might then be viewed as not desirable by the conscious mind, so ambivalence/stuckness has you in its grip. No amount of external pressure works. Even determination just increases the stuckness, so action is equalled by reaction. Unconscious desires for body shape are generated to achieve the perceived goal of being slim. This thought is embedded and has been constantly reinforced, meaning *WUTUB*: slim.

This now unwanted condition may have originated in many ways, including ill-conceived thinking and choices. However, this moment has arrived, and it is now all about change for the future. As with weight loss, the thought, "I don't want to be slim" just appears in the unconscious as, "I want to be slim". Start at a Restore Point by building a phantom world where you feel and visualise being happy and content with a healthy body shape. For a quick boost, recite at a fast, regularly repeated pace, feeling the emotion, "EVERY DAY, IN EVERY WAY, I AM GETTING BIGGER AND BIGGER". This helps deliver the message that you want change. Then construct a goal to see yourself as you desire to be, in surroundings where you would feel contented. Keep coming back to this fantasy because the unconscious will accept what it is given and then help you achieve.

Conception

There is present a powerful desire to have a baby. If pregnancy does not soon follow, this leads to the prevailing thought, "no child". The mind ruminates on this desolation and the unconscious contributes to the perception; *WUTUB*: you are childless. It is necessary to get the unconscious heading in the same direction to change the prevailing thoughts. So instead of negatively thinking, "no child", constantly think of children in a positive way. Make plans in your imagination. Keep the thought in bright light and know you are happy. Every time you see children say, "yes" and feel happy. When seeing a child or children around you, never dwell on the emptiness or feel sadness; when you see children playing, feel happy. When couples adopt a pregnancy often follows because the prevailing thought then is positive.

Ageing

The saying, "think young, stay young" is appropriate at this moment. Whatever your ailments, pick out a good time to relax and use the Restore Point exercise. Afterwards, never resign yourself to apathy by not having a goal, be it gardening, holidays, grandchildren or anything else; visualise yourself being involved, make plans and don't just accept life.

Exercises

Eyesight

The eyes are muscles and need exercising, and there are several techniques available for free on the Internet. I also recommend using Emotional Freedom Techniques (EFT) exercises or the easy alternative at a quick repeated pace, feeling the emotion, "EVERY DAY, IN EVERY WAY, MY EYESIGHT IS GETTING BETTER AND BETTER". Do this while exercising the eyes.

Hair

Hair restoring ads claim rubbing in cream restores hair, while science says you need to change your diet to improve hair health. By understanding the process described, these options could be successful if while shampooing you say with conviction, at a quick repeated pace, feeling the emotion, "EVERY DAY, IN EVERY WAY, MY HAIR IS GETTING LONGER AND LONGER". Look in the mirror each day and say, feeling pleased, "it is growing great!"

Posture

People take walking for granted and accept it by saying, "this is how I walk". But it can, and often should, be changed, particularly because adopting a correct walking posture can remove back problems and straighten rounded shoulders. If you look at well-balanced athletes, dancers and martial artists, their feet appear to glide; they are heel-toeing gently, which keeps them well-balanced and upright, ready to move in any direction. I suggest to clients to make walking a form of meditation. Do not walk with the head leading; we are an upright species, so walk from the hips, with the abdomen forward, then concentrate on small steps while saying, "HEEL, TOE, RELAX". When this becomes normal, the body assumes a better posture.

During the time of writing this book, I was twice asked for help by people with shopping trolleys who were incapacitated because of a severe back spasm. To avoid this, rather than dragging trolleys start pushing them from chest area; having head and shoulders slumped over the trolley is a recipe for a bad back. It is better to keep upright, walk as though waltzing with the trolley, heel-toeing, and adjust the handle to a good height. If you feel you need a walking aid, do not guess at what to use; seek professional help to stop any structural damage. The saying, "use it or lose it" is sound advice because any bad habits in a muscular movement become an unconscious desire.

Post-Stroke Recovery

This involves improvement and compensation; time is only a great healer after an argument, not after a stroke. Plasticity, the ability of the body to compensate, never ends. It is the fight with ambivalence and stuckness that is difficult. After a stroke it is what had been considered normal, the automatic actions, that frequently disappears. Motivation is key after a stroke as plasticity occurs through the action of building new neural pathways. *WUTUB* is vital in making the best of the new circumstances, and goals are very important. Have a major goal to make the best recovery. The task ahead can seem massive and daunting, so break the steps down into individual tasks. Learn everything possible about what is necessary to achieve goals, then practice. If this is difficult, keep visualising the stage. See yourself being successful, keep repeating the visualisation and as the unconscious starts relearning it will gradually respond. The more the body changes the easier it becomes to make changes and overcome the ambivalence.

Becoming a Controlled Moderate Drinker

This is going to be difficult unless it really is a desire. I try not to be dogmatic with clients, always aware that if you take a "big brother" attitude the action-reaction to this is for people to increase their drinking. Many well-meaning people try to get others to stop drinking using threats or coercion.

The pleasure that you felt when first drinking alcohol turns against you; that feeling as you thought, "I really enjoyed that" was the alcohol quickly entering your bloodstream, removing all feelings of anxiety and stopping you caring about anything as you became stress free. Following this comes looking forward to repeating this feeling of not caring. Alcohol was endowed with a power, and then reached a time when no amount was enough.

I advise everyone to first start with a period of abstinence, as much for health reasons as anything else, and get ready to have a minimum two or three days dry each week before regularly having long intervals of abstinence to know you are in charge. In this way, you are preparing the unconscious for the change from alcohol having a prominent position in your life. If you knew the consequences of drinking without control when you started, what would your choice be now when contemplating drinking alcohol for a second time? From now on, intelligence makes the choice.

There are compelling health and cognitive reasons for moderation. I recommend people who take charge of their lives to drink in line with recommended alcohol unit guidelines. The two-drink maximum is an excellent self-imposed rule. One drink reduces anxiety and the second adds to the feeling of being relaxed. This though is as good as it gets. After the second drink, the "cognitive you" is under threat, and drinking is now dangerous. Drink more and your intelligence disappears and alcohol and the imagination take over. Anything can occur as you are no longer in charge and no longer care how much you consume. All the excuses to drink more are readily generated from your imagination and have been well-prepared and repeated many times. After two drinks, would you want to trust your whole life to this dissolute being? That is what you do regularly. The alcohol did all the good it can do in two drinks, and it goes downhill after that. The reason to stop at this point is to keep your intelligence in charge at all times. In this way you will achieve all your life goals, not just talk about them in an alcoholic haze.

Visualise, as with weight loss, a picture of yourself knowing you are healthy and successful. By having a goal your unconscious will help by not generating desires at old trigger situations. Whenever entering into a situation when you will be drinking, always have a plan. See in your mind the "healthy you" leaving, feeling happy. This is key to staying in control. Always make a plan for any situation with the goal of beating the repeated desire for more alcohol. The first time you do this is the start of the journey to good health. In addition, read again about Thought Stopping and how to use it to help you sleep.

A soft drink, or a lower alcohol shandy or spritzer, helps keep the units in check, keeping the "I really need a drink" thought at bay. Prepare in advance a visualisation of you achieving your goal. If you are going to be in a situation for a longer spell, plan how you will drink. You can mix soft drinks and periods not drinking when in company. Telling others what you are doing can be difficult at first, but it becomes supportive in the long term. Clients have often explained that they tested the two-drink line, and all reported that at two-and-a-half drinks the alcohol takes over, and they stop caring.

Cannabis

Clients who want to stop using are usually heavy users, people spending hundreds of pounds each month on cannabis. It is not highly chemically addictive, and I tell clients the chemical reliance can be broken in three or four days; most report back that it took five days. However, the psychological reliance is more difficult to change. This becomes an entire lifestyle, with the user spending a huge amount of time getting the money, organising the best source, the paraphernalia, bongs, spliffs, joints, papers, tobacco, where to use and who with. I feel the main problem is often the level of prominence the drug has been given in a person's life. Many feel it has been the reason they have survived. This is an "imagination thought", and many former heavy users find the technique of Thought Stopping helpful. I feel the nature of the drug makes clients open to meditation techniques.

The main damage is that people who began using regularly at a young age are emotionally immature in their responses whenever they have a problem. Smoking cannabis stops them caring because it prevents them facing up to any stress or anxiety. Using relaxation techniques and behavioural management, I work on ways to change routines. It is not easy, largely because the chemicals in cannabis suppress some hormonal responses. Testosterone gives people extra drive to succeed, but sometimes the "peace, man" stance is an example of heavy users just not caring and being emotionally stuck.

Stop Smoking Tobacco

The chemical nicotine interacts with hormones in the brain. It has powerful effects from the start, while the comfort and pleasure felt when the drug enters the "brain soup" gives psychological power to this highly poisonous drug. We often hear the sighing pleasure of, "that feels good", "I really needed that" or "I am dying for a cigarette". All that hunting around for a place to smoke, all the emotion that gets built into a visualisation in the mind of this most desirous of pleasures, one that has the power to overcome any intellectual knowledge.

For the smoker, the amount of pleasure you thought you received is proportional to the power you have invested in the drug to run your life. You have invested immense power into a substance that took only three or four cigarettes to establish itself. Perhaps you thought it made you look cool. These days, people often wean themselves off the chemical addiction with patches, gum or sheer willpower. People sometimes go months or more without smoking, then in a moment their defences drop and they start again. This is not a chemical reaction, it is a psychological one. You invested all that power in a cigarette. Reading about relapse prevention can help, and you can practice Thought Stopping in advance. There will be difficult moments, so it is good to be prepared and stay in charge. Say to yourself when approaching difficult times, "I CAN DO THIS", and you will. Your intellect, not your imagination, is in control.

Sport

While there is a need for physical attributes, which many people could naturally possess, other processes are also involved in being successful. Thinking and thought processes are often discussed as part of the visualisation techniques used in all professional sports. The following is a way to take charge of motivation to help achieve your desire.

Repeat visualisation actions many times. This has the same benefit for skill as physical practice, building muscle memory and the autonomic nervous system reaction. Wanting to be successful can in itself leave people stuck; the desire mixed with doubt can leave no clear map for the unconscious, and development stalls. Practice physically and keep repeating the exercises. Understand all the actions involved in a move and the body will learn the skill. Keep practising your skills; practise visualisation of the techniques then at the moment the sport starts in earnest the intellect must step sideways. When in action there is no time to think. In fact, thinking becomes a hindrance and must be turned off. High-level table tennis should not be possible as it is so fast there is no time to think. Martial artists know it as "the zone", as do ball hitters; the moment when everything appears to slow down.

Self-talk can be very counter-productive here. As explained, the unconscious cannot picture a negative so the zone can be breached by the thought, "I must not miss". The only command then understood by the unconscious is "miss". If when taking a golf shot you visualise a hazard, you hit what you visualise; so the only visualisation should be a successful shot. In the build up to a match, anxiety can become prevalent, fear is overriding and stalling occurs. Do not leave the mind ruminating on maybes and uncertainties in the build-up; there should only be one decisive thought. See yourself finishing the match, being successful, and feel the celebration as well. The focus on the successful completion of the task has to be the goal; not a goal made up of uncertainties, just a picture and feeling of success with no fudging of the unconscious

With Thought Stopping we can only have one thought at any one time. When watching sport, look at place kickers as an example. See them rehearsing every movement in their mind and feeling and knowing they are going to be successful. Top golfers visualise every shot, going through all the movements knowing the golf ball has cleared a hazard and landed on the green. Once ready for action, thinking must stop. Concentrate quickly on something else and let the action take place on its own. Your body, from all the practice, knows what to do, so don't stop it. To assist with this, put your thumb and forefinger into an "O" shape;

concentrate on this action and let the body react, or put a smile on your face thinking about it. Let your body do its work; don't undermine all your practice by thinking at that pivotal moment, as you can either hit or miss if you have the wrong thoughts. Rehearse in your mind then turn the mind off. For example, for a potential goal scorer at a corner; as the kicker prepares don't get distracted, visualise while saying, "I can head the ball down into net", then concentrate, smile or put your fingers in an "O", and let the action happen.

How to be Successful

The goal can be anything, any kind of fantasy. Just repeat what you want to yourself while ruminating on the goal. The processes in our development are not always successful; no preferences, no luck involved. If there is no clear fantasy goal, life will be full of inconsistency. It is only our conscious judgement that defines failure. This could occur if a dysfunctional lifestyle or the use of substances negates any earlier life goals, leaving only the expectancy of failure and a feeling of drifting through life.

What society considers deviant or perverted behaviour by a sex offender are actions described as acting out or living their fantasies. Saddam Hussein's biographies describe how his stepfather had used him from an early age as a human scarecrow to keep pests from crops by killing them. A large, strong, clever boy, he became a conniving bully who annihilated people along the path to success. In this way, he dispensed with any distractions from achieving his goal. This is synonymous with the process described in development by *WUTUB*. The unconscious has no preferences and no intelligence; it constructs our world in line with our mentally dramatised desires, our fantasies. Every person has arrived at his or her goal by having a fantasised desire. The more successful, the more the goal is singularly and passionately craved. This includes politicians, leaders in industry, headline actors, star musicians, indeed any kind of success. Sport, arts, business; the list is endless. All success is derived first from fantasy, which then enables singularity when following the map.

It works because the only desires generated by the unconscious are ones that are positive in attaining the goal. Any negative influences to divert from this are ignored, and unless there is some kind of unforeseen trauma, the outcome will be successful. Sometimes life, through unconscious choices, has meant following a path of dysfunction or is too mundane. As stated earlier, there is no blame attached to how you arrived at being You. If you want to change and define your own future, you need to understand the processes involved in how you evolved to be You; then you can use this same process to decide on your own goals and maps to achievement. This is not age related; to many people, success is money or stature, and to others it relates to contentment with themselves. I have explained this process to many people and found that changes occurred when they started living life according to their own desire and no longer tried to conform to what they thought would please others.

Summary

Steps Towards Change

- It must be attainable and include an emotional desire to live the goal

- Be willing to work to gain the ability to focus singularly

- Start learning to differentiate between your intellect and your imagination

- Practice catching the imagination's repeated responses to situations; notice the triggers then make decisions

- Check your emotional state, and as previously described use intelligence to make choices

- When there is a goal, past-embedded triggers will distract you at first; they must be stopped or dissipated so that you don't respond to them

These procedures promote motivation. Gradually, as successfully being in control is emotionally appreciated, the taking charge of thoughts becomes automatic and your unconscious will be able to aid you in your goal.

Chapter Six

THE BIGGER PICTURE

The process of development has a variety of outcomes, with many traps for disadvantaged people. As has been explained, from birth we naturally look outside ourselves for sustenance and try to please to survive whilst vying for attention. At this point there are no choices with regards the influences that affect our decision-making. We copy our family and our local society in an effort to be accepted, and we can then, through blinkered choices, follow any path and react to attempts to coerce us onto a different path. As we have seen, the choices are made not by our intellect but by our imagination's emotional fantasies. If left to our own decisions, our personal life journey could be positive and successful, or viewed by society as negative and/or antisocial. Life becomes about surviving and accepting.

These then are our choices. Others though have learned to control our decisions to meet their own agendas. These people use persuasive techniques that are not focused on your intelligence to influence your decision-making. The subject of their personal agendas is presented to arouse an emotional response and leave you with only one choice, which is for the persuader's benefit or to fit their preferred agenda. Master persuaders include conmen, salesmen, politicians, clergy, gurus, advertisers, spin-doctors, newspaper editorials, sexual predators, employment bureaus and those who lure people into sexual or domestic servitude. The offerings may be beneficial or not; however, they are proposed in a way to circumvent your intellect in examining their offerings.

There is an endless list of people in society with individual agendas to influence others' lives.

The inner belief that our needs are maintained exclusively by external sources keeps people trapped in their particular situation, even if related to psychological or physical health. Stuckness keeps people in every life circumstance looking outside themselves for assistance. The reality is that your life has been built from your choices; the problem can be that you have not made intellectualised decisions when coming up with those choices.

GPs have skills to help patients when there is something organically or physically wrong. A problem arises when an illness is considered psychological or psychosomatic. Medication is expected or even demanded by patients, but the reality is that the events are only taking place in the patients' heads. Despite this, they want and expect medication. When working with clients referred for a substance abuse problem, I have regularly encountered those who have had a long-standing medical prescription. It is not unusual for medication to be prescribed for more than twenty years. One client, while listing her daily medication, said the chemist had explained that if she had to purchase the prescriptions herself the cost would be about £250 a month. The client had been referred for her alcohol consumption, and the amount of medication she was prescribed was proof to her of a serious illness. There was nothing physically wrong with the client; she had an extremely controlling mother, which caused her to respond with extreme reactions. Medication, or the use of substances, cannot help in these kinds of situations. In therapy, we cannot change the cause but we can assist the client to change the way they react to, for example, emotional bullying.

I have included this client example as a lead-in to an alternative action. This would involve a doctor directly addressing a patient with psychological symptoms during the first consultation, explaining, "this is one of those thinking things you have learnt about and is often talked about. You need to change your thoughts. If you need any further help I can get someone to explain it to you". I have found myself with clients telling me all about the tests they had undergone and how the doctors were mystified. This leaves me to explain that I imagine the doctor felt unable to say the cause could be psychosomatic. The causing event could have long ceased, but the illness originally was protracted and the symptoms, whether physical or psychological, became stuck. Personally, I would look carefully at any illness that involves the immune system because I have found this closely follows our personal emotional fantasies about the prevailing condition. Our unconscious produces for us what we fantasise about, and the more stress involved the stronger the outcome: *WUTUB*.

Drug & Alcohol Rehab

As with normal life, substance abuse rehabilitation generally follows the basic belief that help and ultimate success arrives from external sources; a belief in help from higher beings or re-education.

As you will now understand, the process described in this work involves clients taking charge of their own lives and self-determining their own futures. Many people do not have a belief system, and others react to what they perceive as probably well-intentioned people bullying them all their lives. There is success in these programs, but also a high failure rate with clients who are unable to commit. Individual therapy and workshops can act as guides to show how to take charge. Investing power in the individual, and not in a chemical source, means they are no longer empowering external forces to control their lives. It is about enabling people to take charge of their substance misuse by employing their intelligence, meaning their imagination no longer controls their lives.

I facilitated a workshop with four participants for an hour a week over five weeks. The participants were three Class-A drug users and one long-term heavy alcohol user. All had experiences of detox and rehabilitation in the past that they had been unable to sustain. I outlined the process involved in putting their intelligence in charge, and from the third session onwards no one used words such as "if", "but" or "maybe". In their own time, unasked or prompted, outside of the group each member developed their own plan and strategies for their own lives, having practised

Thought Stopping, understanding the process that enabled them to take charge of their lives. Their intellect could then gain ascendency and strategies to work on their behaviour could begin. Self-defeating thoughts, negative ruminating and irrational beliefs cause stress in people's lives. Stopping them changes a life.

Most people are not aware of the power of their thoughts. Uncontrolled thinking produces emotional responses, increasing anxiety and stress. People benefit from working within a group, as facilitated learning enables them to take charge of their own lives by understanding the process. Groups help with understanding and this then provides motivation, and people often understand more clearly when they work with a subject in a group. While some manage on their own in therapy, others find that group sessions help. The group brings several minds to bear on a problem and enables people to recognise that others can struggle, increasing the chances that a productive idea will develop. When a member hears an idea from the group, he or she sees the idea in the context of intense thought about a problem, which enhances the process. Usually, an idea is only partly formed when it arrives. People have the potential to emotionally feel and thus learn from an idea they first encounter in a group, and these insights tend to last.

In my therapy, I have not encountered clients who were unable to work towards taking charge of their own lives; instead they feel empowered by deciding their own destiny. This is usually the first time in their lives that they have made a goal for their own benefit, no longer seeking to please others. They want to achieve for themselves.

The Big Picture: Changing Society

Young peoples' unconscious is the controller of development in every context. These days, people are inundated with mainly unachievable images that are perceived as ever-changing goals, meaning life for many becomes banal. Life's significance is drowned out by external stimuli, and importance is placed on celebrity and possessions. The enormity of this fantasy world infects the unconscious, which then generates desire viewed as the emotional mood of that moment. We can only have one thought at any one time, and these images of the unachievable, if ruminated on, promote dysfunction and an unreachable goal for the unconscious.

From birth, our needs are all met externally; to certain degrees some people do not overcome the need to be the good child and earn praise, and this thought pattern causes much stress. People who are successful are generally self-sufficient. As explained, what others think about us cannot and does not have any meaning in our personal evolution. Our unconscious develops from our personal and individual emotional fantasy goals. Without specific maps with which to achieve success, fruitful life development is in abeyance. So bombarding children with the media's perception of what is required to be successful – to possess items and have a life they feel others would envy – makes things very difficult. A life of external gloss, no substance, solely desiring celebrity; people are responding unconsciously to society's banal brainwashing.

In life, they can question events and start to realise and

understand the processes involved and that they themselves are forming their whole world. This would negate them going through life thinking that others are thinking about them and the corresponding thought that others have power over them. In education, in areas of deprivation, positive role models are not in the ascendency. Rather than fantasying about others, by understanding the processes involved young people could set their own goals and then begin fantasising about being successful themselves. From a young age, the difference between intelligence and fantasy could be explained, together with how to use their imagination as the precursor for advancing their intelligence. They then, in pre-adolescence, could be primed to ask the crucial question of themselves: "Is this intelligence or is it my imagination?"

With an understanding of how we develop they could then choose to become the person they decide to be, not what others might want them to be or find themselves forced into limited choices by local conditions. With this understanding, doctors could then say to patients, "this could be a thinking thing", and respond to a person delivering an extremist view with the thought, "this person has addicted thinking". The following is offered as a hypothesis of how this could be achieved.

The belief that everything we desire comes from outside sources has continued since childhood.

In infancy, all needs are presumed to be supplied by others, a belief that some kind of fulfilment comes from how others view us. The reality is that this thinking keeps adults stuck in acceptance and taking the easy option; guessing, then often following manipulative people who capitalise on the desire of an infant to "be a good child" and to "belong". External circumstances in life are always going to create differences. Those who experience a privileged childhood, with its advantages of being healthier, feeling safer and a better education, galvanise feelings of being special and then *WUTUB*; they may become successful in life thanks to events and beliefs generated by imaginative thoughts. People *become* superior because they *think* they are special. The polar opposite of this special imagined position is one of survival, for example, living in a suburban jungle blighted by poverty, crime and violence. What can people become while fighting deprivation?

Any combination of events can shape the imagination in a negative or positive fashion; choices made while young are the result of decisions imposed by circumstances, and then the unconscious, primed by the imagination, guides these burgeoning lives to succeed in their surroundings. But it could be different. Instead of leaving children's lives to the vagaries of their surrounding culture, we could show them how to use their intelligence and their imagination. By their creating satisfying psychological lives we could even level out the playing field, as each child would learn how to make better choices to map out their futures. From a young age, children would need to understand the difference between imagination and intelligence, and this could be integrated into subjects during development so that goal setting could be incorporated later, again through felicitation and not imposed.

Children are being taught integrated subjects, such

as mathematics and art and design, at a suitable stage. It could be explained that they are using their intellect and imagination and making decisions and choices regarding the subject – using their intellect by combining the senses – and thereby controlling the outcome or goal using both imagination and theory. A history teacher asking, "What was he thinking when he did that?" about a historical figure; in literature, an author's thoughts about a character, or a poet's about their poetry; in science, imagine taking a trip on an exploding atom across the universe and seeing cells develop into life. All of this is in the imagination, but requires intelligence to work out the possibilities.

In critical studies, see and discuss the different ways spin is used to direct the imagination without intelligence being involved, and determine how others are trying to exert control and influence over, for example, the items we purchase. Understand reasons for goal setting and the importance of the choices we make. For example, picture a person using substances. Observe the gratified feeling, then the possible reactions to this originating action. It would be better in education for young people to understand the processes involved in development; when presented with a statement they can decide whether this it is a statement of fact or of fantasy from someone's imagination.

Examine how successful people have constructed goals. What is important is what they think about their own self. If a child has been forced to exist in dysfunctional way, understanding this process will help them lead a better life. It is not about being told what to achieve and the best ways to live. What they need to learn is how to achieve it. They can do this by understanding and being in charge of their own life, which enables them to live a productive life in society.

The imagination has been the precursor for society in art, design, agriculture, science, engineering and much more, but it is the intelligence that delivers the finished product. Our imagination is the sense that has been the precursor for wars, genocide and all manner of other senseless, selfish acts. The paranoid thoughts of religious extremists have caused thousands of years of conflicts. Imagine how different debates and discussions would be if all were based on facts. If, from an early age, individuals understood which sense is the intellect and which is the imagination, it would eradicate many problems and reduce the immense financial and emotional cost to our society.

I say to clients who have changed their lives and worry they may regress to previous thinking patterns: "If you escape a burning house, you don't go back in". When you take charge of your life, you do not regress, creating a stuckness that is then beneficial.

When choices and decisions are made using our intellect, as has been described, success is the result. Trouble occurs when a person indulges their imagination, believing their thoughts to be real and unwittingly defining their life. This indulging of the imagination can be magnified by societies, causing a mass psychosis.

The means to counteract this is to heighten the ability of people to differentiate between intellect and the imagination, and train them to make their own decisions. Experience has shown me that people respond by making healthy decisions when the repetitive thoughts from the past are dissipated by understanding the process of thought generation. Making intellectual and not emotional decisions and choices means lives are then governed by facts not fantasy, and *WUTUB*. We are then able to enjoy the products derived from the imagination and the intellect in harmony.